Rural Extension Handbook

Dr. Vijender Singh
B.V.Sc. & A.H., B.J.C., P.G. (A.W.C.), M.Sc.
Presently APS to Vice President of India
NEW DELHI, India

Prof. (Dr.) M.S. Vasishtha, Ph.D.
Head
Department of Extension
College of Veterinary Science,
BIKANER (Rajasthan) India

International Book Distributing Co.
(Publishing Division)

Published by

INTERNATIONAL BOOK DISTRIBUTING CO.
(Publishing Division)
Khushnuma Complex Basement
7, Meerabai Marg, Lucknow 226 001 U.P. (INDIA)
Tel. : Off. : 2209542 - 45, 4045308, 2450004, 2450007, 2459058,
Fax : 0522-2458629
E-Mail : ibdco@sancharnet.in
E-mail : vijendersingh2005@yahoo.co.in

First Edition 2007

ISBN 81-8189-179-1

Composed & Designed at :

Panacea Computers
2nd Floor, Agarwal Sabha Bhawan, Subhash Mohal
Sadar Cantt., Lucknow-226 002
Phone : 0522-2483312, 9335927082
E-mail : prasgupt@rediffmail.com

Printed at:

Salasar Imaging Systems
C-7/5, Lawrence Road Industrial Area
Delhi - 110 035
Tel. : 011-27185653, 9810064311

PREFACE

Interaction between man and animals has been continuing since time immemorial. Animals are playing an important role in human life. Man is dependent on animals for transportation, agriculture, company, food products and general utility during the course of centuries. While man derives enormous economic benefit from animals, animals receive protection and care from human beings. Our approach to animal rearing and agricultural management has changed according to times. Newer scientific ways have been evolved for rearing, keeping of various animals so that maximum economic benefit is derived in a humane way. This knowledge is very important for those engaged in activities related to animal practices. Hence, the need for a book on Rural Extension was being felt since a long time.

Extension education is an important branch of Agriculture and Veterinary Sciences which has a great bearing on increasing food production, thus raising socio-economic status of rural population. This book deals with various aspects of providing scientific knowledge to the rural population especially about animal husbandry.

I wish to express my gratitude to my Guru Dr. M.S. Vasishtha, Professor, Department of Rural Extension and Education, College of Veterinary Science, Bikaner, Dr. (Mrs.) Chandrakala Sharma, Professor, Surgery Dept., College of Veterinary Science, Bikaner, Dr. Dinesh Rana, Polyclinic Ajmer, my wife, Dr. (Mrs.) Parveen Lata, Dr. Gopal Choudhry, Dr. Ajay Choudhry, Dr. Rajesh Choudhry, Dr. Sanjay Choudhry, Dr. Kuldeep Chehal, Dr. Sunil Choudhry, Dr. Prem Lata, Dr. Narender Kumar Dabas, Dr. Anil Dabas, Prof. (Dr.) Vijender Dabas (Gujarat), Dr. Subhash Dabas, Dr. Vinod Kumar Verma, Dr. Sat Pal Yadav, Dr. Jogender Malik and Shri Akeshwar Prasad, without whose cooperation this book would not have come into existence.

Suggestions and comments will be highly appreciated for further improvement.

Dr. Vijender Singh
Dr. M.S. VVasishtha

PREFACE

Contents

Contents

Chapter 1

Training of the Trainers

Training of the trainers in rural extension work is a key to success in the real sense. Trainers are Change Agents who have been designed as Extension Officers, Subject Matter Specialists, Technical Experts, Field workers and Village Level Workers. In addition to the paid servants, voluntary and active workers, innovators and venturesome people also come forward to cooperate and participate in different extension activities in their area. It is, therefore, necessary to propose different syllabi for different groups that will suit to one's ability and skill. Simultaneously, selection of desired type of trainers at all levels, is extremely essential. Aptitude for such job, rural background, hard working, honest dealing and soft spoken virtues are some of the most important and common demands for such work.

Training

It means to educate a person so as to become skilled, qualified and expert in doing a particular job.

Types of training for Extension Workers

1. Pre-service : It is the training of Extension Workers received before joining actual job, i.e. schooling to professional colleges is called Pre-service.
2. Inservice training : It is the training after joining the service. It includes
   (a) Oriental of extension work.
   (b) Including training about work.

(c) Short term courses.

(d) Job oriented training for special job.

(e) Periodical meeting, symposia, seminars and work-shops.

Training of farmers/community

1. Hold training at a time convenient to the people.
2. One week duration is enough for a course.
3. Venue of course should be suitable for demonstrations.
4. Production-cum-demonstration camps and discussion groups of people of 1 – 2 days duration.
5. Training of rural youth by keeping them in Youth Clubs arranging camps of one week duration : 15-20 in a year.

Adult education

Extension educationalist is needed mostly to educate adults.

Essentials of adult learning

Adults learn for "profit" provided "goal" is clear and they receive "satisfaction" from what they have learnt, seen and tried. Words, spoken or written, are often forgotten.

Learning process

Any change of behaviour which takes place as a result of experience may be called learning. People learn through practice and experience, which emerge out of active participation.

Learning experience

It is a mental or physical reaction to seeing, hearing and doing.

Principles of learning

1. New behaviour helps in satisfying felt needs.

2. Learning should be meaning and one should know why he/she is learning.
3. Learning is prompt when two or more senses are used at a time.
4. Effect of sense on learning rank 1.0 percent through taste, 1.5 percent through touch, 3.5 percent through smell, 11.0 percent through hearing, and 83.0 percent through sight.
5. The learner's ability to learn is 10 percent of what they read, 20 percent of what they hear, 30 percent of what they see, 50 percent of what they talk, and 90 percent of what they say as they do a thing.
6. Learning is effective when learners participate actively and when situations are real and problematic. Learning is facilitated when the learners are ready to learn.
7. Individuals differ in their learning ability.
8. Learning is more effective if it is challenging.
9. Attitude and motivation are important in learning.
10. Methods of instruction affect learning viz. [*a*] telling by teachers or hearing by learners, [*b*] showing by teacher or seeing by learners, and [*c*] telling and showing by teachers or hearing and seeing by learners. When recalled after 3 hours later and 3 days later, the learners remembered [*a*] 70 percent, [*b*] 72 percent and 20 percent, and [*c*] 35 percent and 65 percent, respectively.

Teaching

It directs the learning process. It is a process of creating situation that facilitates learning process.

Lecture notes and lesson plan

The lecture note means storage of information but lesson plan means how to teach it. They should not be confused for each other.

Role of a teacher

To –

1. Present materials
2. Motivate students
3. Make students aware how they are performing

Methods and techniques of teaching

1. Trainee-dominated
    a. Use of Library
    b. Use of Laboratory
    c. Use of questionnaire
    d. Use of survey
    e. Use of field trips and observations
    f. Project to work on
2. Trainer dominated
    a. Lecture
    b. Counselling
    c. Case work
    d. Demonstration
3. Cooperative
    a. Apprenticeship
    b. Group discussion, i.e. seminar, symposium, panel etc.
4. Functional :- Developing skill and ability to do, i.e. operating machine, film projector etc.

Principles of teaching

1. Purpose of course should be clear
2. Desire of students to learn
3. Students be allowed to ask what they do not know precisely
4. Favourable and appropriate physical conditions
5. Participation with curiosity for learning

6. To use experience of learners
7. Teacher must prepare well (both lecture material and the equipment needed)
8. Method of instruction varied and appropriate
9. Teacher is always a learner
10. Good teacher and learner relation is essential

Qualities of a good teacher

1. Up-to-date in his subject
2. Thorougly prepared
3. Interest in students
4. Fair in dealings
5. Clarity of expression
6. Not satisfied with poor performance
7. Likeable
8. Alert and perceptive
9. Experienced
10. Encourages and motivates students

Steps in process of teaching

1. Securing attention of learners
2. Developing interest in learners
3. Creating desire to learn
4. Inspiring conviction in learners, i.e. asking the learners to take part in surveys and meetings
5. Ensuring action so that learners are in acting mood
6. Maintaining satisfaction by worthwhile practices, honesty and service
7. Developing and holding confidence by sound teaching, demonstrations, pleasant contacts and creating local leaders' interest.

Cone of experience

The cone of experience is a visual device to explain inter-relationship of various types of audio-visual teaching aids as well as their individual position in learning process. As we move from its apex to base, there is increase in directness viz,

1. Verbal symbols
2. Visual symbols, i.e. charts, maps, graphs
3. Radio recording, still pictures
4. Motion pictures
5. Exhibits
6. Field trips
7. Demonstration
8. Dramatic participation
9. Contrived experience i.e. models, mock-up etc.
10. Direct purposeful experience i.e. immediate sensory contacts with reality

Syllabi

Syllabus for Extension Officers

1. Educational psychology
2. Rural sociology
3. Rural extension
4. Audio visual aids
5. Teaching methods in extension
6. Communication methods
7. Programme planning
8. Administration

Syllabus for Subject Matter Specialists

1. Interest
2. Awareness
3. Training

4. Communication
5. Preparation of extension material
6. Audio Visual Aids
7. Participation
8. Demonstration camps
9. Exhibition, Film shows
10. Visits

Syllabus for Field Workers

1. Survey work
2. Technical efficiency
3. Human dealing
4. Maintaining records
5. Reporting

Syllabus for village level workers

1. Human dealing
2. Identification of problems
3. Approach and contact
4. Rapport
5. Reporting

Syllabus for college students

A. Theory

1. History, introduction and earlier attempts in extension
2. Community development and extension education
3. General and specific extension education
4. Rural psychology, socio-economic and agro patterns
5. Communication and teaching methods
6. Cooperative societies
7. Adopter categories and programme planning
8. Diffusion of innovation and transfer of technology

B. Practical

1. Preparation of graphs, pie diagram, histogram, flow chart
2. Charts and tables for normal physiological patterns
3. Photographs, pictures and diagrams depicting improved practices
4. Handling and use of audio visual aids
5. Survey work in selected areas
6. Educating package of practices for adoption
7. Camps, meetings, leaflets, demonstrations and film shows
8. Impact of extension education, its evaluation and recommendations in the form of a paper at the end of the course study.

Qualities of an Extension Worker

He must :

1. identify the problem
2. fix the priorities
3. plan the programme 'Win friends'
4. win friends
5. influence people
6. coordinate the team work
7. communicate
8. receive maximum participation
9. transfer of technology
10. evaluation and reconsideration

Qualities of a Subject Matter Specialist

He must:

1. be through in his subject or the area of specification
2. have defined his package of practice to deal with
3. know how to demonstrate them
4. know how to apply them

5. know the advantages
6. know necessary precautions
7. have a open mind to reconsider
8. be ready to face criticism
9. not be overambitious
10. not be overexciting

Qualities of Field Workers and Extension Supervisors

He must:

1. be aware of rural customs
2. be aware of socio-economic constraints
3. be able to understand problems
4. be skilled
5. be honest and hard working
6. work as a connecting link between his officers and farmers/community or farmers
7. work as one of them in a community or farmers
8. know everyone personally
9. be able to carry on a follow-up routine
10. be confident and correct in his judgement
11. be enthusiastic to speed up activity
12. be courageous to meet difficult situation and should have cooperative habit
13. have a helping and service attitude with an ideal of 'Simple Living and High Thinking"
14. be able to use all extension methods and audio visual aids
15. be able to arrange help from various departments and funds the answer to convey
16. not be impatient so as not to give up, if matters move slowly
17. not press and educate people by instructing
18. not lose sense of humour when overbusy or worried
19. not be unhappy when criticised
20. not become alarmed when people lose maturity and have childish behaviour.

Qualities of a Village Level Worker and Volunteer

He must :

1. be a ruralite
2. approach each in a community
3. be in perfect rapport
4. not belong to any group
5. have his fellowmen
6. respect his seniors
7. report immediately and correctly
8. help in all possible ways
9. not escape from his duties
10. not make blind excuses and should overcome superstitions.

Qualities of an Extension Administrator

He must have :

1. integrity
2. faith
3. sound judgement
4. health
5. sense of purpose of direction
6. technical soundness
7. decisiveness, quick and correct decisions
8. fairness
9. courage
10. initiative
11. perseverance
12. versatility
13. expression power
14. sense of honour
15. organisation sensitivity.

Chapter **2**

Teaching Extension

A. EXTENSION EDUCATION

The term "EXTENSION EDUCATION" combines the adult education and informal education. Give a man a fish, he will eat for a day, but if we teach him fishing and he starts to fish then he can go on eating fish for ever.

Definitions

According to Douglas Ensminger : It is education to change the attitude of the people with whom work is done.

According to Kelsey and Hearne : It is an out-of-school education in which people learn by doing.

According to V.T. Krishnamachary : It is a continuous process designed to make the rural people aware of their problems, ways and means by which they can solve them; inspiring them towards positive action in doing.

According to O.P. Dahama : It is formal and informal education assisting people to bring about continous improvement in their socio-economic status. He defines that Agricultural Extension Education is a two-way process where the problems of client system are brought by change agents for finding solution in institutions or laboratories, and the results are taken in the acceptable form by the change agents to the client system.

In our opinion : According to M.S. Vasishtha and Dr. Vijender Singh : Veterinary and Animal Science Extension Education is propagation of approved practices and techonology in the field by lawful agencies for increasing food production, energy and products of animal origin to meet local and export demands so as to establish a stable animal husbandry-industrial economy.

Objectives of extension teaching

1. General : For farm, home, village etc. should aim at rapid increase in skill, health, education, crops, livestock etc.
2. Specific : Should aim to –
    a. change outlook of people,
    b. develop responsible leadership, village organisation and village institutions,
    c. improve practices and methods for increased production,
    d. increase rural industry for increased income and employment,
    e. motivate families for betterment,
    f. upgrade social status of village,
    g. cut down high cost and toll.

Principles of extension teaching

It should :-

1. be based on needs felt
2. be according to local conditions
3. start with people as they are
4. be according to democratic procedures
5. start for simple problems first and then for difficult ones
6. give maximum benefit to greater number of people
7. be made in consultation with client system through their leaders and organisation
8. be based on the principles of helping people to help themselves
9. be adjusted on the basis of feedback from the people, and

10. be clear to every body

Psychology of extension teaching

The psychology of science of mental life. Educational psychology deals with acts as they are. Psychology as applied to extension is concerned with behaviour psychology which includes educational, industrial and religious psychology.

Scope of extension teaching

To fill up gap (need) between what is (actual situation) and what ought to be, is the scope of extension teaching as a method in the process of community development. It implies to all the fields whatsoever, viz. agriculture, animal husbandry, home, education, health, business etc.

Characteristics of extension

It is :

1. cooperative
2. educational
3. teaching
4. informal
5. flexible
6. broad in scope
7. family centered, and
8. voluntary

Concepts of extension teaching

There are following five elements in sequence concepts of extension teaching :

1. Situation and problem
2. Objects of solution
3. Teaching and plan of work
4. Evaluation, and
5. Reconsideration

Extension process

It includes :

1. helping people to help themselves
2. enabling the people for learning by doing, seeing and then believing, recognizing felt needs and how to work
3. developing an individual, village leader and client system
4. backing of extension workers, technical staff and Subject Matter Specialists
5. establishing rapport and guiding by extension worker, and
6. motivating for applying science outside the organized class room.

Extension Worker versus Community Development Worker

Extension worker deals with the technical subject matter to introduce desired change in the client system whereas community development worker deals with sociological and economic aspects of introduced change depending on data and observations. Extension education and community organisation are two methods of community development.

Role of an Extension Worker

He has to :

1. conduct survey
2. use most appropriate extension methods
3. create group leadership
4. improve rural life, environment and economy
5. propagate improved practices and methods
6. organize people
7. part knowledge in rural masses
8. act as change agent in the extension process
9. introduce desired changes in behaviour of the client system, and

10. draw resources from people, government and universities for extension programmes.

B. TEACHING METHODS IN EXTENSION

Extension teaching is an art. The process requires skill, patience and experience to educate the masses. Extension education is an informal training and out of school teaching where people learn by doing. It is something very difficult from class room teaching where resident instructions are learnt and reproduced at regular intervals. Continuing education imparts awareness, desire, satisfaction, trial and action. In the course of such training, change agents and client system form a two way channel of working to find solution of the problems to make a comfortable living. The complexity of entire system lies in variety of client system and the different methods of teaching. Teaching methods therefore comprise work. Families with whom the extension work has been done draw more benefits than those with whom extension work has not been done.

Classification

The teaching methods in extension can be classified in two ways, i.e. 1. According to methods of approaches and 2. According to their forms.

Teaching methods according to method of approaches

These can be classified as (1) Direct Approach or contact, and (2) Indirect Approach. The Direct Approach can be (a) Group approach, and (b) Mass approach. The Indirect Approach is through local leaders. On an average seven out of eight families change behaviour by direct contacts.

The individual approach could be through face to face contact, personal visits, letters, telephone calls, farm and home visits, and office and hospital calls. A person is best tackled by individual approach.

The Mass approach could be by bringing information to a great number of people through films and exhibitions, radio talks, televised programmes, recorded talks and handouts.

Teaching methods according to their forms

These can be classified as (1) Spoken, (2) Written, and (3) Visuals and Audio-visuals.

Spoken

a) Meeting of all kinds, i.e. for method conducting and result demonstration involving black board, charts, audio-visual aids, movie etc.

b) Farm and home visits

c) Office and hospital calls

d) Telephone calls

e) Radio, tape recorder, gramophone records.

Written

a) Pamphlets

b) Leaflets

c) Bulletins

d) News stories, news, wall newspaper

e) Personal letters

f) Circular letters

g) Books

h) Articles in magazines, journals and newspapers

i) Writing for radio talk.

Visuals and Audio-visuals

a) Methods demonstration

b) Result demonstration

c) Exhibits

d) Posters

e) Black board, charts, slides. Film strips, photographs, flannel graphs and other visuals

f) Motion pictures

g) Television

Demonstrations

These are mainly of two types, i.e. (1) Method Demonstration and (2) Result Demonstration.

1. The method demonstration is a short time demonstration given before a group to show how to do in a better way an old practice or an entirely new practice. This method is not concerned with proving the worth of a practice but only with how to do something.

2. The result demonstration is a mean of communication where the results of a new method are compared with the results of the traditional method and thus the superiority of the new method is proved and established.

Audio-visual aids

These are classified as (a) Visual Aids, (b) Audio Aids and (C) Audio-visual Aids.

A. **The Visual Aids are further classified as** (1) Non-Projected Visual Aids, and (2) Projected Visual Aids.

The Non Projected visual aids are of two types, i.e. (1) Teaching Type and (2) Display Type

The Teaching Type visual aids are:-

a) Chalk board or blackboard

b) Picture including photographs and hand drawn pictures

c) Flash Cards : These are the series of cards, when presented in sequence tell a complete story

d) Flip Book : It is similar to a set of flash cards but it is pictorial and bound at the top in the form of calendar, i.e. it is a picture book

e) Flip Chart : A few charts on a picture theme put together and bound together at the top

f) Flannel Graph or Felt Board : This is a board with surface of felt, flannel or "Khaddar" cloth material on the back of which there is sand paper to stick

g) Bulletin Board : A board with background of coloured cloth which can be either a plane board or closed one with glasses or netting etc. for displaying news sheets, announcements, booklets, bulletins, circular letters, newspaper cuttings, cartoons, pictures, charts, posters, maps, graphs, subject outlines etc.

h) Exhibitions : Exhibits, models, stand, framers etc.

The Display Type visual aids are:-

a. Posters

b. Diagrams of machine, building, person, animal, crop or any required object

c. Diagrams in the form of charts that contain series of ideas and can be of several types like pictorial chart for how to do the things

d. Organisational charts to show structure of an organization from head to the lowest rank.

e. Flow chart for showing series of processes to obtain a result and to tell a story how a product is obtained

f. Tree or stream chart to show divisions and sub-divisions represented by a trunk of trees with branches and sub-branches or stream (river) with its tributaries and sub-tributaries

g. Suspense chart or Strip Tease chart for depicting full story in writing or in a picture and is kept covered with strips of paper. As we talk we remove the strips one by one

h. Time chart or Table chart in tabular form

i. Graphs representing the date, i.e. line graph, area graph, bar graph, multiple bar graph, divided bar graph, pie graph, and picot graph. In picot graph use actual symbols or figures to indicate the proportion amountas given in numerical table, i.e. milk bottles regarding quality of milk, animals or man for their population, bags for wheat or fertilizer etc.

The Projected Visual Aids are classified depending on types of projection, i.e (1) Direct Projection, (2) Indirect Projection and (3) Reflected Projection.

(1) Slide projector either manual or automatic, film strip projector and film projector come under is called Direct Projection type of visual aids.

(2) Overhead projector is an example of indirect projection type of visual aids.

(3) Opaque projector or epidiascope is reflected projection type of visual aids.

B. The Audio Aids are either (1) Recording Type or (2) Non-Recording Type.

1. There are three ways of recording sound. i.e. (1) Mechanical, (2) Magnetic process, and (3) Optical process. Examples of recording type audio aids are (a) for mechanical : record player with discs to play, gramophone, (b) for magnetic : tape recorder, ferrograph, and (c) for optic : sound recording, on movie film.
2. Examples of Nonrecording type audio aids are radio sets, telephone, wireless set, intercom, and public address equipment comprising microphone, amplifier, loudspeaker, earphone, headphone operated either by battery or electric power.

C. The Audio-Visual Aids are

(1) Projected Type, and (2) Non-Projected Type

(1) The Projected type audio visual aids are talkies (films with sound) or feature films, documentary films and television etc.

(2) The Non-projected type audio-visual aids are puppets, drama, folk songs and dances.

Meetings

There are several type of meetings, viz.

1. **Direct contact** : With individuals or groups. On campus or farm visits.
2. **Field days** : For general objective of extension education.
3. **Camps and campaigns :** for specific objective at a time.
4. **General Meeting** : To meet many people.
5. **Forum** : Special type of meeting to invite viewpoints from the floor of house observing the time limit.
6. **Round Table** : Subject centred discussion of facts sitting around a table led by someone. Maximum number of members is 20.
7. **Seminar** : It is like round table but opinions based on facts are discussed.
8. **Symposium** : It is a conference in which several aspects of a non-controversial subject are presented by several persons.
9. **Conference** : It is a meeting for consultation of any organization, usually as an annual feature.
10. **Panel Discussion** : six to eight persons are selected for depth and diversity of understanding a subject with a capable chairman as presiding officer. They sit in front of an audience and discuss the subject in controversial manner but with raised voices for 40-50 minutes so that the audience may hear the discussion. It is followed by a discussion by audience for about 40-50 minutes. No body makes a speech and discussion is over when the interest is at the pitch.
11. **Group Discussion** : Six to twelve persons as a group are given equal rights, privileges and opportunities to discuss a problem.
12. **Workshop** : A special type of working conference for professional improvement and for inservice training.

13. **Tours** : Mostly educational ones.
14. **Congress** : Formal meeting of delegates for discussion and coming together.
15. **Convention** : It is a formal assembly.

Journalism and Literature

1. **Leaflet** :

It is a single sheet of new or specific information on a single topic and when leaflets are folded it is called folder.

2. **Pamphlet** :

It is a booklet dealing with number of related topics consisting of two or more sheets, stitched together and not bound.

3. **Bulletin** :

It is an official report of public news and may deal with a number of related topics.

4. **Circular Letter** :

It is a letter containing general information sent to a large number of people periodically or on special occasion.

5. **Newspaper** :

May be daily or periodical with news-type or service-type information.

6. **Film shows**
7. **Exhibitions**
8. **Fairs**

Relative influence of methods on adoption of improved practices

Methods influence each

I. Indirect by influencing local leaders highest : About 20%

II. Method demonstration, general meeting, higher : About 10-16%

Farm visit, news story

III. Result demonstration, bulletin, office call high : About 6-7 %

IV. Circular letter low : About 2%

V. Correspondence radio talk, lower : About 1%

VI. Poster, exhibit, telephone call, lowest : Less than 1% study course

Chapter **3**

Diffusion of Innovations in Community

Diffusion of innovations in community is done by communication. The communication is a conscious attempt to share information, ideas, attitude etc. Thus it is a two-way process involving the extension worker and the community. The communication is a process of social interaction and helps in approach (contact) for effective extension work.

To define, community is a group of people living in a geographical region depending on each other for their needs and bound in a particular social system.

According to U.N.O., community development is a process by which efforts of the people are united by those of the Government authorities for improving their socio-economic status.

Building community organization and teaching extension education are two methods of community development. The community organizations are (1) farmers organization, (2) women organization, and (3) youth organization. The village organization like "Panchayat" in India, cooperative and school, are three basic institutions that should be made effective in community development work making committees at village, block and district levels.

Components of social structure of community are (1) institutions viz. Government, family, religion, education, and economic system, (2) groups, (3) organizations already mentioned above, (4) pattern of influence, viz. caste, wealth, ability, reliability etc, (5) valuesystem viz, truthfulness, honesty etc, (6) communication media.

Concepts of community development work are (1) "Self determination: for the proposed change, (2) "will to change"' (3) "community pace" for carrying on several works, and (4) "growth in capacity" of community to deal with future problems by developing problem solving techniques.

Community Development Process means (1) establishing rapport, (2) identifying problems and needs. i.e. appraising the situation, (3) programme and projects and long-term projects, (4) selection of initial projects and long-term projects, (5) securing participation and involving people, (6) developing effective communication channel, (7) development and use of community organizations, and (8) developing community leadership.

Limitations of Community Development are (1) traditional society, i.e. old ways and practices, resistance in early stage, (2) illiteracy, (3) lack of communication channels an specific mass media, i.e. television, radio sets, broadcasting stations, roads, automobiles etc., (4) limited staff, (5) people with vested interests who befool the people. e.g. quacks, (6) insufficient number of properly trained workers capable of introducing change in the community who are mostly outsiders, and (7) public criticism for failure of the programme due to any of the reasons mentioned above.

The Community Development Programme is weak when (1) programme is largely a Government administered one and not a people's programme with assistance from Government agencies, (2) there is emphasis on achieving target figure or end results and less emphasis on social change (change in attitude) by not using correct methods and practices, (3) lack of understanding of objectives , (4) lack of confidence of people in government machinery and in the programme as a whole, (5) extension education methods which are so essential for democratic approach, remain mostly as claim, (6) lack of uniform understanding about concept, principles, methods, role, functions etc. from village to national level, (7) lack of proper and adequate supervision and guidance both technical and administrative at various levels, (8) lack of democratic leadership to replace autocratic authority, and (9) workers feel unhappy at all levels because their moral is not very high and the unhappy workers or change agents cannot make a good organization.

The community development programme should be integrative type, i.e. countrywide in scope. The impact of the programme on community results in the form of (1) awareness of the programme (2) communication with outside world, (3) institutional development, and (4) leadership development.

Success or failure of the community development programme depends on (1) physical and (2) cultural factors. The physical factors include physical, natural and man-made resources. The cultural factors include attitude of people, habits, traditions and beliefs.

Innovation

Innovation is an idea perceived as new by the individual.

Diffusion

Diffusion is a process by which an innovation spreads. This diffusion is a communication between two persons or organizations out of which, one knows about innovation and another yet does not know.

Elements of diffusion

The elements of diffusion of an innovation include (1) innovation and (2) its communication from one individual to another (3) in a social system (4) over time.

Characteristic of innovation

1. **Relative advantage** : That new idea is superior to others.
2. **Compatibility** : That new idea is compatibility with cultural norms.

3. **Complexity** : Degree to which the innovation is relatively difficult to understand and use.
4. **divisibility** : Degree to which the innovation may be tried on a limited basis.
5. **communicability** : Degree to which the results of the innovation may be diffused to others.

Inventors

These are the persons who create new ideas. Innovators are not necessarily the same persons as inventors.

Deviation

It is defined as departure from a social system norm.

Opinion leaders

Individuals who are influential in approving or disapproving new ideas.

Communication

Communication must always be in the medium of instruction officially and constitutionallyrecognized in the state and the local language is called communication.

According to J. Paul League, communication is a process by which two or more people exchange ideas, feelings or impression in ways that each could gain a common understanding of the message. Thus it is an act of getting sender of information tuned to receiver (both ways).

According to Schramn, communication is to establish commonness when two corresponding system coupled through one or more non-corresponding system assume identical status.

According to Loomis and Beegle, it is a process by which information, decisions and directions pass through a social system and ways in which knowledge, opinion and attitudes are formed and modified.

According to Warren Weaver, it is a procedure by which an individual communicator transmits stimuli to modify the behaviour of the individuals.

He is of the view that it is a procedure by which one mind can affect another.

Elements of communication

1. Extension Worker or "sender of information" or communicator.
2. "Message" or content.
3. "Treatment of message" by communicator so that it is clear and understandable.
4. Channels of communication.
5. Receiver of information or audience or communicates, and
6. Response of receiver or audience.

Communication problems

1. Expression of the communicator,
2. Interpretation by receiver, and
3. Response of the receiver.

Scope of communication

About 10-11 hours are spent daily by an individual to communicate verbally. Gesture, facial expressions, movements of arms etc. make communication more effective. People communicate on many levels, for many reasons, with many people, and in many ways. Communication is used in management, education and extension service. Markets of professional communicators are advertisements, newspapers, magazines, journals, oratory and photography. Market needs are continuously increasing for advertising, public relations, radio, television, films and audio-visual experts. There is big scope of communication for improving management and removing time lag. The need for communication has given rise to communication industry.

Model of communication process

1. **Aristotle's model** : It has three elements or ingredients. In sequence, these are
   1. Speaker
   2. Speech, and
   3. Audience.

   Its example is face to face situation of direct communication.

2. **Shammon Weaver's model** : It has got five elements. In sequence these are
   1. Source
   2. Transmitter
   3. Signal
   4. Receiver, and
   5. Destination

   If source is speaker, if signal is speech, and if destination is listener then we have Aristotle's model plus two more ingredients. The transmitter sendsout the message and receiver catches the message for distance.

3. **Westley and Machean's model** : It has also got four elements. In sequence these are
   1. Sender
   2. Encoder
   3. Decoder, and
   4. Receiver

   The sender encodes the message and then message is passed through a channel. The message is then decoded and its meaning is drawn after which the message is clear to receiver.

4. **Berlo's model** : It has five elements. In sequence these are
   1. Source
   2. Encoder

3. Message
4. Channel
5. Decoder, and Receiver.

5. **Leagan's model** : It has got six elements. In sequence these are
   1. Communicator
   2. Message
   3. Channel
   4. Treatment of message
   5. Audience, and
   6. Response of audience

The response of audience is very important to bring about change in people and hence the Leagan's model of communication is considered as best in extension work.

Facotrs affecting dissemination of information

Effective dissemination of information on improved practices requires.

1. Well trained extension agents, i.e. local leaders, subject matter specialists and extension workers.
2. Motivation of extensionagents so that they may work with zeal, enthusiasm and high morale.
3. Approach of extension agents to (1) understand problems, culture and resources of client system, (2) motivate the client system to adopt improved practices, and (4) evaluate the work.

Model is a result of events and experiences, i.e. cheerful, optimistic, gloomy, and recentful. Sentiments are directed towards specific object of persons like love and hate. The moods and sentiments are expressions of emotions. When feelings become intense, we have emotions. The emotions have a tendency to persist in the forms of moods and anxiety. The anxiety is some kind of persisting fear. Love for a subject of teaching may be aroused by various stimuli like method of teaching, inspiration from the teacher or extension worker or leader, and content of course etc.

Importance of emotions in teaching extension is (1) to arouse emotions of people for making teaching interested, (2) once emotional, people will do extraordinary things, (3) strong emotions will break up undesirable emotions, (4) emotions are strong motivating forces of action, and (5) emotions are to be given due consideration.

Motivation is a process of initiating a conscious and purposeful action. Bodily needs, personal wants, emotions, feelings, attitude, situation or objective environment, habit and will to improve status and place in society are motives that motivates someone. Experience or activity isevaluated between pleasant and unpleasant. If pleasant, the person has attitude of approach to that experience otherwise his attitude is of withdrawal. Once a habit is established, it requires only a stimulus to set it in action. The people act differently in different situations. Objective environment is a set or readiness to respond in a particular way. If needs are met with, a person is satisfied otherwise he is frustrated. There is universal tendency to improve status and place in society. Motivation for extension work is very important. The villagers as well as extension workers must be motivated for the success. Awards, incentives and recognition help in motivation, learning and teaching.

Natural opposition to change, sects, agriculture, religion, standing, conflict between families passing through generations and problems in group living are some very important points in rural psychology.

Crowd is a gathering of considerable number of persons around a point of common attention. Mob is an active crowd whereas audience is a passive crowd. Mob psychology or behaviour of mob includes (1) mental homogeneity, (2) emotionality, (3) irrationality, (4) diminished sense of responsibility, (5) sense of power, and (6) sense of anonymity.

Propaganda, that is opposite to extension is a systematic attempt by means of mass communications to influence attitudes. It is a technique that can be used either for good purpose or bad. It is ordinarily looked upon as dishonest or misleading. It is based on suggestions. It gives one side or wrong side of the picture. It cannot be verified. It leads to intolerance of free thinking. It is unethical and influence beliefs. It seeks uncritical response. It has no fundamental methods. It has only purpose of conquest of masses.

Chapter **4**

Adoption in the Client System

The CLIENT SYSTEM or social system which is dealt with by extension teaching is a part of the community. "It comprises particular people engaged in particular job, for whom particular type of work is to be done by the extension workers".

Communication is through approach or contacts and it increases the effectiveness of extension work in client system. Every individual has certain aspirations which motivate him to come in contact and participate in extension training. These DESIRES include wish for (1) security to earn and live nicely, (2) response for want of recognition, appreciation and love by the people, (3) recognition by awards and status in society, and (new experience either to gain or to try.

Two or more people in process of communication constitute a GROUP. INSTITUTIONAL GROUPS are family, religion, caste, economic, education, status, age, sex etc. ORGANIZATIONS are formalised groups, systematically arranged units of people with the object of achieving some common goal in which there is specific role of each person.

Any member in a group occupies by virtue of his belonging to a sex, particular age group, birth, marital status, physical abilities, achievements and designated duties. The status is of two types, i.e. (1) ASCRIBED STATUS is there come by birth, and (2) ACHIEVED STATUS which is earned.

Role is part of an individual that is played as a result of his status in the group or society i.e. child or parent, youth or old, leader or follower, literate or illiterate, subordinate or supervisor, husband or wife etc.

A person may not participate in a group for following reasons, viz for (1) fear, (2) insecurity, (3) lack of skill, (4) vested interests, (5) sect, (6) political group, (7) way improper to get the things done, (8) personal demand for special drive, and (9) poor and irregular extension work etc.

Following are the ways in which frustrated individuals adjust to frustration that block their participation in a group, viz.

1. **Aggression** : When someone's ideas are not accepted or are ignored, he may strike back.
2. **Compensation** : One may feel not good in taking and offers to help in other way.
3. **Rationalization** : Thinking that project is of no utility and there is no need for a group.
4. **Identification** : Alliance with a friend thinking that he is always right.
5. **Displacement** : Disliking for the chairman of the meeting and finding faults in the report.
6. **Conversion** : If one's project is not accepted he tries to postpone meetings.
7. **Idealization** : Overestimation of ability of self and friends in a group claiming to be always right.
8. **Projection** : One,fs if wrong, may put blame on some imaginary cause.
9. **Regression** : Majority prefers to go with crown because they seldom get their way, and
10. **Pending complaints.**

Change agents

The change agents are (1) Voluntary local leaders, and (2) Professional personnel i.e village level workers and subject matter specialists etc.

Local leaders

A local leader is a person who initiates action and coordinates activities which help the client system to adopt improved practices. There are several types of leaders i.e. (1) hereditary, (2) occupational, (3) personal because of knowledge and skill (volunteer), (4) political, (5)social and religious.

A leader can be identified by (1) discussion method, (2) workshop method, (3) questionnaire or socio-metric method, and (4) seniority and past experience.

Following are the methods to develop desire for the change in a leader, (1) to create awareness by showing them new practices and their results, (2) arrange tours to demonstrate and show work of progressive persons, (3) evaluate results of new practices and present these to teach them, and (4) arrange their consultations with the Subject Matter Specialists.

Methods of training leaders are (1) informal and (2) formal. The informal methods include observation in the field and work of others, reading literature and circular letters, and talking to other leaders and progressive persons in the client system. The formal methods include lecture, discussion, forum, panel, symposium, audio-visual aids, field trips, apprenticeship (learning things by staying with others who adopted improved practices), training groups or camps, direct assistance from expert, buzz groups (discussion in all groups of less then seven persons for small duration of about 6 minutes), and giving responsibility to local leaders for developing confidence in them.

Adoption of improved practices

Adoption of improved practices in client system starts with the diffusion of innovations, i.e communication.

Adoption process is the mental process through which an individual passes from first hearing about an innovation to final adoption, i.e.

1. Learning theory
2. Decision making, and
3. Adoption or rejection

Stages of adoption are

1. Awareness
2. Interest
3. Evaluation
4. Trial, and
5. Adoption.

Length (period) and rate of adoption vary from an innovation to another and adopter categories.

Following are the characteristics of adoption viz.

1. **Rate of adoption** : It is the relative speed with which the innovation is adopted by members of client system. It is usually measured by the length of time required for a certain percentage of members for the client system to adopt an innovation.
2. **Profitability versus compatibility** : A controversy
3. **Interaction effect**: It is the process through which individuals in a client system who have adopted an innovation influence those who have not yet adopted.
4. **Overadoption** : It occurs when an individual adopts a new idea under conditions when experts would consider him irrational to do so. Rationality is the use of the most effective means to reach a given end.

Adopter categories in the client system

Adopter categories according to time of adoption of an innovation are

Ist Innovators 2.5%

2nd Early adopters 13.5%

3rd Early majority 34.0 %

4th Late majority 34.0 %

5th Laggards 16.0%

Characteristics of adopter categories

I. Innovators :

1. Venturesome, i.e. accept risk
2. Young in age
3. Highest social status
4. Largest and more specialized operation
5. Wealthy
6. Closest contact with scientific information sources
7. Interaction with other innovators
8. Relatively greater use of impersonal sources
9. Some opinion leadership
10. Very cosmopolitan

II. Early adopters

1. Respect, i.e. regarded by many others as a role model
2. High social status
3. Large and specialized operation
4. Greatest contact with local change agents
5. Greatest opinion leadership of any category in most social systems and client system
6. Very localite

III. Early majority

1. Deliberate, i.e. willing to consider innovations only after peers have adopted
2. Social status above average
3. Average size operation
4. Considerable contact with change agents and early

adopters

5. Some opinion leadership

IV. Late majority

1. Skeptical, i.e. overwhelming pressure from peers needed before adoption occurs
2. Social status below average
3. Small operation
4. Little specialization
5. Small income
6. Secure ideas from peers who are mainly late majority or early majority
7. Little opinion leadership

V. Laggards

1. Traditional, i.e. oriented to the past
2. Little specialization
3. Social status lowest
4. Smallest operation
5. Lowest income
6. Oldest
7. Neighbours, friends and relatives with similar values are main information source
8. Very little opinion leadership
9. Semi isolates change in adopter categories over time

There is a considerable shifting of individuals in a client system from one adopter category to another over time. The laggards are most likely to drop out of the client system.

Role of adopters and rejectors in the client system

There are active and passive roles of adopters and rejectors in the client system. Some adopters are active in influencing other individuals to adopt. Others, after their own adoption decision, play a passive role in spreading an innovation. Rejectors of an innovation may also be active or passive in communicating their opinion about an innovation to their peers. The active rejectors may also be opinion leaders influencing others in the client system not to adopt the improved practice

Chapter 5

Planning and Impact of Extension Programmes

Planning of extension programmes is a procedure of working with the people in an effort to recognize unsatisfactory situation or problems and determine possible solutions or objectives. It is a conscious effort to meet the needs, interests and wants of people for whom the programme is intended. In planning an extension programme, planners are required to know where they are and what they ought to achieve, so that they may better judge what to do and how to do it. Thus it is an intentional effort carefully designed to attain certain specific and predetermined objectives. It involves (1) a study and use of facts and principles, (2) knowledge, imagination and reasoning ability, (4) skill and research techniques, and (5) ability to synthesise facts and value judgments in a process of sound decision making about objectives.

Components of planning for an extension programme are

(1) people,

(2) needs and interest of the people

(3) useful technology

(4) educational process

(5) analyzing situations

(6) making decisions about what should be done

(7) determining useful action and

(8) projecting the desired shape of things in future

Need is felt for developing extension programmes because

of –

(1) poor and affluent societies

(2) problems created by inequalities

(3) economic inequalities mixed up with racial inequalities

(4) poor nations in the world, and

(5) influence of world powers and cold war due to foreign aids.

Basic principles of planning the extension programmes are

(1) clear and significant objectives

(2) planning at top and lower level

(3) crucial questions taken into consideration

(4) general agreement among various levels, i.e. village, block, district, state and nation

(5) programme be based on adequate current facts pertaining to local, regional, and national situations

(6) most significant needs should receive major attention

(7) skillful involvement of progressive village leaders

(8) long period plans are more effective

(9) integrated approach to problems of farm, home and community is more sound and effective

(10) cultural values and client system must be taken into account

(11) programme contents must be determined with care and preciseness, and

(12) interpretation of the programmes to officials, non-officials and people.

The extension programmes are of three types, i.e.

1. Integrated type : Countrywide in scope
2. Adaptive type : Self help efforts by client system
3. Project type : Limited to a region only

Essentials of an extension programme are

(1) planning with and not for the people
(2) indispensable use of local leadership in developing and executing the programme
(3) programme be based on facts
(4) programme should be useful, of high interest and profitable
(5) programme planning requires time
(6) one must hold big idea foremost in the attention of people
(7) habits, customs and culture of people must be given due consideration
(8) use of local material in planning and development
(9) programme should be cooperative having group action, group support, community wide awareness of its meaning and purpose and
(10) to avoid waste of money, time and energy

Abilities needed by a planner of extension programmes are

(1) to understand nature and role of extension service organization
(2) knowledge and understanding of technology related to subjects concerned with the programme
(3) clear objective in guiding and execution of the programme
(4) to arrange inputs and organize people
(5) skill in human relations
(6) skill to develop relationship between principle and practice, and
(7) skill in nicely dealing with inquiries and complaints without hampering and extension programme

There are three approaches in programme building i.e.

(1) Autocratic approach
(2) Laissez-faire approach and
(3) Democratic approach

(I) In Autocratic approach, a person or a small group attempts to regulate activities of others largely through his choosing.

(II) In Laissez-faire approach, a person regulates activities of others on the line that "if you ever want any help, let me know". This might be called "Cafeteria style" or "filling station" plan or service without extension which does not result in most effective programme. Two things in this type of approach are never settled: who is the leader and what the leader's influence.

(III) There must be democratic approach in building the extension programmes. Soundest programme results when ideas of members of the client system, i.e. laymen are involved. What the extension workers and specialists think, is incorporated into the programme. The people need time to change their minds, and time to make up their minds to change. The change people and the extension workers are to build the programme.

The plan of work is an outline of activities, so arranged as to enable execution of the entire extension programme. Calendar of work is a plan of work arranged chronologically for a calendar year and that too mostly monthwise.

Following are the steps in sequence in developing programme for extension work, etc.

1. Study the situation, i.e. people, habits, attitude, values, physical conditions like livestock, home, health, education etc. and all background information.
2. Set up a planning committee.
3. Identify local leaders and obtain their support.
4. Determine needs of the people and solutions of their problems.
5. Setting up of objectives for all processes.
6. System of priority to the felt needs.
7. Workout teaching objectives and teaching methods.
8. Carryout the programme.

9. Evaluate and determine the reconsideration of plan for setting up revised objectives.
10. Periodic review of the situation and reconsideration of plan for setting up revised objectives.

The official organizations involved in planning of the extension programmes in India at (a) national, (b) state, (c) district, (d) block, and (e) village levels are (1) Minister, (2) State Directors, (3) District officers, (4) Block Development Officers, and (5) village level workers, respectively. Similarly, nonofficial organizations at these levels are (1) Central committed, (2) State Development Committee, (3) Zila Parishad, (4) Panchayat Samiti, and (5) Gram Panchayat, respectively.

Target is a mark to which the work is to be completed quantitatively in a given time.

Reports are records of past, mirrors of present and charts of future as written statements for all activities and achievements. Essentials of a report are (1) accuracy, (2) thoroughness, (3) conciseness, (4) proper emphasis, (5) attractive appearance, and (6) better if on pro-forma for the standardized form and records. Types of reports are (1) daily, (2) weekly, (3) fortnightly, (4) monthly, (5) quarterly, (6) half yearly, and (7) annual.

Records are all files and registers necessary to be maintained for each type of operation or functioning.

Unique programmes of extension education in India:

Year	**Programme**
1888	Land Improvement Loans Act
1904	Cooperative Act
1908	Tagore's Youth Organisation in Kaligram
1921	Tagore's Rural Reconstruction Institute in Shriniketan
1933	Gurgaon Rural Reconstruction
1934	Rural Reconstruction Phori and Poona

1935 Christian Missions
1936 Gandhian Construction Programme
1945 Indian Village Service
1946 Firka Development Scheme of Madras State
1947 Etawah Pilot Project
1948 Nilokheri Experiment
1951 1st Five Year Plan
1953 Ministry of Community Development
1958 Intensive Agriculture District Programme

Rajpur Package Programme

Extension Programmes in Blocks:

(1) Small Farmers' Development Agency [SFDA]
(2) Marginal Farmer and Agriculture Labourers (MFAL)
(3) Integrated Rural Development Programme (IRDP)
(4) Command Area Development (CAD)
(5) Desert Development Programme (DDP)
(6) District Development Agency (DDA)
(7) Agricultural Universities
(8) Agriculture Research Station (ARS)
(9) Krishi Vigyan Kendra (KVK)
(10) Krishi Gyan Kendra (KGK)
(11) Farmers' Training Centre (FTC)
(12) Tractor Training Centre (TTC)
(13) Training of Youth for Self Employment (TRYSEM)
(14) National Bank of Agricultural and Rural Development (NABARD),
(15) Adult Education
(16) Lab to Land
(17) New 20-point Economic Programme etc.

On the recommendations of Planning Commission, the Central Ministry of Food and Agriculture commends the extension work in India through (1) Indian Council of Agriculture Research (ICAR) and (2) State Department. The directives of ICAR follow a channel, i.e. University, Directors extension education, extension wing (KVK, KGK, FTC), Subject Matter Specialists and village level workers. The directives of Directors follow a separate channel, i.e. Block Development Officers (BDO), Extension Officers of different departments, and village level workers.

Impact of extension education

Impact of extension education ina client system is judged on every individual and group.It is a numerical figure obtained on dividing practices adopted by the total practices. Thus by avoiding losses the indirect economic gains can be roughly calculated on the ground of practice adopted. This figure plus direct gains us a figure for total benefit.

After carrying out extension programmes, these are evaluated to determine progress. The evaluation is an analysis of relative merit or demerit of persons, groups, programmes, situations, methods, materials, processes, and changes etc. The terms 'appraisal' and 'measurement' can be used as synonymous for evaluation.

Reconsideration of each step of the extension programmes carried out must be done periodically in consultation with the members of the client system so that if needed the plan of work be modified for better effort to achieve the goal in a desired period.

Chapter **6**

ASOSA & ECPPA System of Extension Education

Affluent Save Our Souls Approach & Effluent Complete Package of Practices adoption system of extension Education

(For Rapid Socio Economic Development)

By running an S.O.S. (Save Our Souls) help centre on the campus for sheep husbandrymen around the year, following the diffusion of innovations in the field as well as by conducting veterinary and animal husbandry extension work in the rural areas for several years, it was found that there exists yet another unidentified and most effective method of extension education. It has been named later as ASOSA & ECPPA System of Extension Education", unlike other systems which are named first, and then implemented and worked out. It is "Affluent S.O.S. Approach and Effluent Complete Package of Practices Adoption". It is complete package of practices in sequence which are made understandable to the persons to whom the extension services are rendered. With the lapse of desired time the demonstrable results of the S.O.S. help are appreciated by the member of the client system who adopt at least single innovation (improved practice). He then further adopts the complete package of practices as devised by the Subject Matter Specialist, thus completing the ECPPA part of this system.

Though process is initially slow because of the client system approach, but it steadily achieves the desired goals. It is the most practical system by which downtrodden rural masses can be definitely lifted to progress in a country like ours and other under developed and developing countries. It suits best for traditional and orthodox community as well as all the scientific subjcets particularly biological sciences viz. medical, veterinary, agriculture and animal husbandry etc. The members of the client system must be dependent for their livelihood mainly adopted or their need must be so much important that if the technical help in the form of extension service and extension education is not extended, the member suffers tremendous losses in future. Extension education is the most important constituent of the ECPPA part.

There is a need for fixing the technology and improved practices for their propagation and not the targets which is the beauty of this system because the extension programme originates from the administrative high ups. That is why, whatever is done is a solid piece of work and result oriented one. Further, even when inputs are not available with the extension agency, the extension programme fairly runs smoothly. Inputs can be polled from sister agencies too. In addition there is not much need for keeping experimental, training and demonstration plots, farms, subjects and objects because units on which work is conducted for rendering the extension services and education belong to the members of the client system themselves. They learn at their own cost for their own betterment. Thus it is rather an inexpensive system of extension education. The only main things needed to run the programme in this system thus are technical expertise alongwith limited but essential inputs and diffusion of innovations through communication. The mystery of success of this sytem is that the members of the client system actively participate in both the ASOSA and ECPPA parts initially to save themselves from crisis followed by adoption of improved practices for better future.

In other words this system may also be called as "Vasishtha'& Singh's Forcep System of Extension Education" in which one arm of the forcep is constituted by the active approach by the member of the client system for S.O.S. help and another by extension education and service which leads to adoption of improved practices by him. Both joined at a point where there is a pool of technical expertise. The forcep may hold one member of the client system, some families, village, block, district, state nation or globe i.e, the system remaining same its operational dimension may increase to any extent. The ASOSA arm (part) may already exist but the forcep is never completed if ECPPA arm (part) is not developed which should be realized for steady progress of masses, states and the nation. The system is most suitable for rapid socio-economic growth.

This system has been established well by us and is recommended for its adoption particularly in all THIRD WORLD countries for speeding up their development. One is to start in each needy occupational unit and each needy family. Do justice and technically contribute your maximum to the prosperity of poor masses in making the whole world happy. When socio-economic status in each occupational unit and of each family is improved, it automatically leads to sound national and international economy. Sincerity is a must in this endeavour and Vasishtha's & Singh system of extension education for rapid soico-economic development is a key to the success. This system also leads a path to the "Gandhian" thoughts. It helps in checking unemployment and flow of rural people to urban areas in search of jobs.

Chapter 7

Cooperative Movement

Contributed by URMUL-Bikaner, Rajasthan Cooperative Dairy Federation

Aims and Objectives of Cooperation

The word "cooperative" means any institution or organization in which people join voluntarily to gain and share the economic benefits while enjoying the equal status, keeping in view the voice of "ONE FOR ALL AND ALL FOR ONE". There is simultaneous development of economic and social status in the cooperative sector.

Mr. Robert Oven of England during the revolution between capitalists and industrial labourers in the period from the year 1750 to 1850 felt and suggested that only cooperative methods can avoid such a competition. The ideas of Mr. Robert and Dr. William King were appreciated and followed by industrial labourers to form the societies and the principles were formulated to include open membership, democratic control, share contribution and to work in set bye-laws.

Philosophy of cooperative

The following aspects were felt to be adopted in institutions or organizations in the cooperative set-up:-

1. University
2. Unity
3. Liberty
4. Fraternity

5. Equality
6. Justice
7. Economy
8. Democracy
9. Education

As such, besides the economic benefit, cooperative organizations have much to do with social benefits for their members shortening the gap between producers and consumers as one of the important end results, thereby eliminating middle agencies in dealing with any business. Urban and rural based cooperatives deal with production as well as consumer societies.

Structure of Cooperative

Mostly the structure of cooperative is federal with two or three tiers. Primary or the basic unit of cooperative sector is organized in democratic form in which interests of beneficiaries are kept in mind according to economic and social status. The legislature is formed to cover the mass population.

A cooperative society is formed by the members contributing equal and nominal share capital. Thereafter the bye-laws, aims and principles of the society are framed and it is registered by the Registrar, Cooperative or State Community.

There may be various types of cooperative sectors like Agricultural Cash Credit Societies, Land Reform Cash Credit Societies, Agricultural Product Marketing Societies and Consumer Societies etc. Likewise every cooperative sector has got its own fundamental principles, aims and structure duly constituted by State, Central or Federal Government. The rule and principles are supported by Cooperative Acts of the state.

A committee appointed by the International Cooperative Congress under the Chairmanship of Professor D.G. Kurvey at Bormouth in the year 1963 submitted its report. The structure and principles of cooperative societies accepted by the member participating countries, i.e. India, England, Germany, USA and

USSR are as under:-

1. Voluntary membership
2. Democratic membership
3. Limited interest on capital
4. Cooperative education
5. Growth of mutual cooperation among the cooperatives
6. Equal distribution of responsibilities and surplus benefits

The cooperative societies formed at initial level are registered by the Registrar Cooperatives of State Government in any sector of cooperation under the set principles and acts. This type of basic cooperative society is placed in category A. A number of such type of cooperative societies will from an "Apex Body", the Category B, in which certain financing agencies and state nominees are the members. Each category of the cooperative societies has certain bye-laws and will form the Advisory Management Committee to look after the work for implementing the programme in the interest of the members.

In India, the cooperative movement started in south in the year 1882 where the cooperative societies were registered under the companies act. Later on shortcomings of the act were remedied by enacting Cooperative Societies Act, 1912. It was also emphasized that State Legislation must maintain uniformity in framing the acts of cooperative movement.

An Imperial Committee on Cooperative was appointed by the Government of India in the year 1915. The Committee visualizsed a four-tier cooperative credit structure consisting of Primary Societies at village level, Cooperative Unions at tehsil level, Central Cooperative Bank at district level, and Provincial State Level Cooperatives.

Chapter 8

Sociology and Psychology

A. SOCIOLOGY

"Sociology" is science of society. To study the social relationship is its subject matter. Group and group mobilization are essential in extension work.

Elements of rural sociology

1. Rural structure
2. Rural social organisation
3. Characteristic of rural life
4. Rural problems
5. Rural moral teaching
6. Rural social life
7. Rural reconstruction
8. Culture
9. Casteism : Upper, backward, scheduled and tribe
10. Personality : Contrast between rural and urban life

"Personality" is an end product of our habit system. What a person conceives of himself is "self" known as personality.

Process of self-development

1. Hereditary
2. Physical or geographical environment
3. Culture
4. Unique experience

Social values

1. Importance of ascribed status
2. Recognition of inequality
3. Patrilinial tendency
4. Status of women
5. Greater male dominance
6. Adherence to well regulated sex relations
7. Charity
8. Tendency of non-violence
9. Respect for old age and elders
10. Religious attitude

Formation of social values

1. Norms
2. Formal and informal education
3. Social change
4. Scientific and technological change

Desired new social values

1. Acquired status
2. Equality for all
3. Modification in marriage norms
4. Charitable disposition
5. Attitude for non-violence
6. Respect for old and elders and consideration for young generation
7. Religion and technology

Social control

It helps in maintenance of desired social value which is called social control.

Agents of social control

1. Gossip
2. Rumour
3. Ridicule
4. Public opinion
5. Custom
6. Tradition
7. Law
8. Social institution

Welfare organizations

1. **National** :
   a. Government
   b. University
   c. Voluntary
2. **International** :
   a. World Health Oraganisation (WHO)
   b. United Nations Educational Scientific and Cultural Organisation (UNESCO)
   c. United Nations International Emergency Fund (UNIED)
   d. Food and Agriculture Organisation (FAO) etc.

Amenities and services for rural development

1. Education
2. Water supply and sanitation
3. Health and medical facilities
4. Utilization of leisure
5. Recreation

Social organization

It is functioning of various institutes in accordance with

their implied purpose. It is dependent on social structure.

Social structure

It is a particular arrangement of interrelated institutions, agencies and social patterns as well as the social status and role which each person assumes in the society or group.

Social process in dynamic society

1. Communication
2. Conflict : Conscious opposition
3. Competition : Struggle
4. Accommodation : Mutual adjustment
5. Assimilation : Adjustment to the changing social scene

Social disorganization

1. Individual disorganization
2. Family disorganization
3. Community disorganization : Political, social, cultural or religious

Social action

1. Idea initiation
2. Legitimization
3. Organization and planning
4. Action.

B. PSYCHOLOGY :

According to William James, "psychology" is science of mental life.

Aims of psychology

1. Environmental adjustment
2. Group behaviour
3. Improvement in environment

Problem of psychology

1. To understand characteristics of behaviour
2. To analyse behaviour
3. To interpret or find meaning of analysis

Characteristic of behaviour

1. Sensing
2. Perceiving
3. Thinking
4. Feeling
5. Willingness
6. Doing

Concept of man according to psychology

1. He is an organism
2. He is able to adjust himself to environment
3. He desires self-preservation
4. He desires race preservation
5. He has learning capacity
6. He thinks

For psychology man is provided with

1. A receiving mechanism, which includes all sense organs, i.e. eye, ear, nose, tongue and skin
2. A connecting mechanism, i.e. brain and nerves
3. A responding mechanism, i.e. glands and muscles

Contribution of psychology

1. Information about personality of people
2. Emphasis on ability and attitude
3. Possibility of guiding the people
4. Behavioural changes with age and experience

5. Information on level of intelligence
6. Information about individual difference
7. Knowledge about psycho-analysis of problematic man
8. Knowledge about sense experience, learning, thinking, aptitudes, inclination and interests
9. Knowledge about stages of development and achievements to prepare future programmes
10. Information on causes of feeble minded persons and other drawbacks. Persons who behave differently are mentally sick and need sympathy and proper treatment from extension workers.

Role of human mind

1. Cognition : Attention, sensation, perception, imagination, memory, conception, judgement and reasoning.
2. Conation : Inherited tendencies like reflexes, instincts and general tendencies like habit and character.
3. Affection : Feelings, emotions, moods and sentiments.

Intelligence

Intelligence is a product of heredity, environment and opportunities to learn. It is inherited capacity as modified by maturation accounts for a greater part of individual variability. It is the ability of an individual to cope with his environment or to adjust himself to the conditions that arise in the environment. Intelligence is organization of abilities to learn.

Areas of intelligence

1. **Abstract ability** : With ideas as in language, words, numbers, science, mathematics etc. professional people are high in abstract ability.
2. **Mechanical ability** : Understanding things in skill trades.
3. **Social ability** : Understanding persons and mixing with people.

Nature of intelligence

1. **Monarchic (Unifocal)** :- One great power of mind dominating over others. Persons who perform all tasks very well.
2. **Oligarchic (multifocal)** :- Persons who perform one task very well but fail to do so in other tasks.
3. **Anarchic (Non-focal)** :- Average of all energies is intelligence.
4. **Eclectic (Two factor theory)** :- According to this theory, the intelligence is that ability of mind which is a combination of two factors 'g' and 's'. The 'g' is general factor and 's' is the specific factor. The 'g' factor is gifted and never changes in a man. The 's' factor doffers in the same man from test to test.

Factors affecting intelligence

1. Hereditary and environment
2. Age
3. Health and physical development
4. Sex
5. Race
6. Culture
7. Social and economic conditions

Measurement of intelligence

1. "Standard-BinetScales for measuring general intelligence". Objective type of tests for different age groups. After conducting the test I.Q. is determined for 4 years, 13 years and adult age groups.

$$I.Q. = \frac{M.A. \times 100}{C.A.}$$

I.Q. - Intelligence quotient

M.A. - Mental Age (needed age for a task)

C.A. - Chronological Age

The level of intelligence may be indicated as follows:-

I.Q.	CATEGORY
0-25	Idiot
25-50	Imbecile
50-70	Moron
70-80	Border line
80-90	Low normal
90-110	Normal
110-120	Superior
120-140	Very superior

140 and over near genius

2. **"Wechsler-Bellevue Scale"** : It is designed for adults. There are two types of tests, (1) Verbal, arithmetic, reasoning, general information, comprehension, memory, span of digits and vocabulary, (2) To arrange 16 cubes in different 7 designs printed on cards. These do not yield M.A. but I.Q. can be determined keeping average I.Q. for each level as 100.

Tests for special abilities

Aptitudes are special abilities in such areas as agriculture and animal husbandry. Following tests have been designed to test the aptitudes

Minnesota Paper Form Board: This consists of 2 dimensional diagrams cut into separate parts. There are 5 figures in each diagram with lines indicating different shapes out of which they are made. One figure is to be chosen that is composed of exact parts of previously prepared diagrams.

Interest tests: Distinguish between real and superficial interests. These tests are more helpful in measurement of motivation than ability.

These can be :-

(a) "**Strong Vocational Interest Bank**" : This is a questionnaire of 420 items to indicate whether one likes, dislikes or indifferent to the activity named. It includes name of occupations, hobbies and personal traits etc.

(b) "**Duder Preference Record**" : This is score for types of occupational areas. Pin punch is done on left of one of the 3 activities that one likes most and to the right of one of the activity that one likes least. Pin punches makes a pattern on understanding sheet from which examiner can count the area. The scores are finally translated from a table into percentage.

Speed or Reaction

It is the time taken by a person to perceive and report.

Reaction time

It is the time that elapses between occurrence of a stimulus and the beginning of a response. It is the way of measuring reaction. It is measured by chronoscope.

Personality test

It is used for measuring more general traits of personality. Measure the dominance, sociability, irritability and suspiciousness. Observe face to face every day or by questionnaire.

Emotional states

1. Anger
2. Fear
3. Joy
4. Surprise

5. Disgust
6. Grief

Influencing people

1. Effective speaking
2. suggestions
3. Creating suitable conditions
4. Technique of influencing :
   (a) Sympathetic induction of attitudes
   (b) 'Yes' techniques, i.e. once a person starts saying yes, he goes on doing so
   (c) Use of newness
   (d) Recognise limitations
   (e) Need-based advice
   (f) Making appeals vivid by using visual aids
   (g) Remove deficiencies of others to arouse their latent

Psychological concepts for extension work

1) Arouse emotion of the members of the client system
2) Motivate them
3) Help in development of an individual
4) Use senses provided to human beings
5) Attention and perception
6) Thinking
7) Communication
8) Group processes
9) Problems in group living

Extension in rural India

There are 0.58 million villages in India to which scientific and technical knowledge is being made available through extension education. More than 65 per cent people in India are living in villages and thus extension education in rural India is of utmost importance. The present monograph "Rural Extension" will be of immense value in this endeavour for all the three aspects of extension, i.e. extension education, extension training and extension service. According to M.K. Gandhi, India can progress only if its villages are developed. This is also true for the whole of THIRD WORLD.

Index

P

R

S

T

V

W